The Quick and Easy Mediterranean Recipe Guide

Irresistible and On a Budget Recipes Affordable for Beginners

Alison Russell

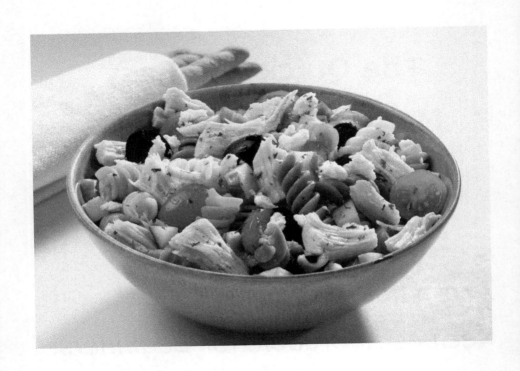

Table of contents

Beans, Grains, and Pastas

Butternut Squash and Zucchini with Penne

Prep time: 15 minutes | Cook time: 30 minutes | Serves 6

1 large zucchini, diced

1 large butternut squash, peeled and diced

1 large yellow onion, chopped

2 tablespoons extra-virgin olive oil

1 teaspoon paprika

½ teaspoon garlic powder

½ teaspoon sea salt

½ teaspoon freshly ground black pepper

1 pound (454 g) whole-grain penne

½ cup dry white wine

2 tablespoons grated Parmesan cheese

1. Preheat the oven to 400ºF (205ºC). Line a baking sheet with aluminum foil.
2. Combine the zucchini, butternut squash, and onion in a large bowl. Drizzle with olive oil and

sprinkle with paprika, garlic powder, salt, and ground black pepper. Toss to coat well.

3. Spread the vegetables in the single layer on the baking sheet, then roast in the preheated oven for 25 minutes or until the vegetables are tender.

4. Meanwhile, bring a pot of water to a boil, then add the penne and cook for 14 minutes or until al dente. Drain the penne through a colander.

5. Transfer ½ cup of roasted vegetables in a food processor, then pour in the dry white wine. Pulse until smooth.

6. Pour the puréed vegetables in a nonstick skillet and cook with penne over medium-high heat for a few minutes to heat through.

7. Transfer the penne with the purée on a large serving plate, then spread the remaining roasted vegetables and Parmesan on top before serving.

Per Serving

calories: 340 | fat: 6.2g | protein: 8.0g | carbs: 66.8g | fiber: 9.1g | sodium: 297mg

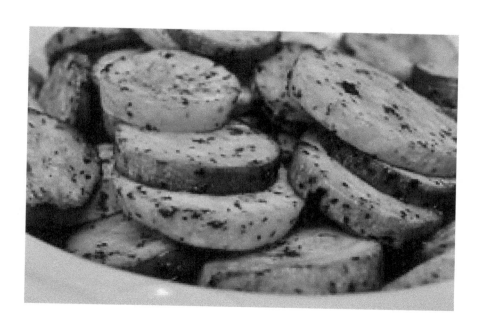

Small Pasta and Beans Pot

Prep time: 20 minutes | Cook time: 15 minutes | Serves 2 to 4

1 pound (454 g) small whole wheat pasta

1 (14.5-ounce / 411-g) can diced tomatoes, juice reserved

1 (15-ounce / 425-g) can cannellini beans, drained and rinsed

2 tablespoons no-salt-added tomato paste

1 red or yellow bell pepper, chopped

1 yellow onion, chopped

1 tablespoon Italian seasoning mix

3 garlic cloves, minced

¼ teaspoon crushed red pepper flakes, optional

1 tablespoon extra-virgin olive oil

5 cups water

1 bunch kale, stemmed and chopped

½ cup pitted Kalamata olives, chopped

1 cup sliced basil

1. Except for the kale, olives, and basil, combine all the ingredients in a pot. Stir to mix well. Bring to a boil over high heat. Stir constantly.

2. Reduce the heat to medium high and add the kale. Cook for 10 minutes or until the pasta is al dente. Stir constantly.

3. Transfer all of them on a large plate and serve with olives and basil on top.

Per Serving

calories: 357 | fat: 7.6g | protein: 18.2g | carbs: 64.5g | fiber: 10.1g | sodium: 454mg

Swoodles with Almond Butter Sauce

Prep time: 20 minutes | Cook time: 20 minutes | Serves 4

Sauce:

1 garlic clove

1-inch piece fresh ginger, peeled and sliced

¼ cup chopped yellow onion

¾ cup almond butter

1 tablespoon tamari

1 tablespoon raw honey

1 teaspoon paprika

1 tablespoon fresh lemon juice

⅛ teaspoon ground red pepper

Sea salt and ground black pepper, to taste

¼ cup water

Swoodles:

2 large sweet potatoes, spiralized

2 tablespoons coconut oil, melted

Sea salt and ground black pepper, to taste

For Serving:

½ cup fresh parsley, chopped

½ cup thinly sliced scallions

14

Make the Sauce

1. Put the garlic, ginger, and onion in a food processor, then pulse to combine well.
2. Add the almond butter, tamari, honey, paprika, lemon juice, ground red pepper, salt, and black pepper to the food processor. Pulse to combine well. Pour in the water during the pulsing until the mixture is thick and smooth.

Make the Swoodles

3. Preheat the oven to 425ºF (220ºC). Line a baking sheet with parchment paper.
4. Put the spiralized sweet potato in a bowl, then drizzle with olive oil. Toss to coat well. Transfer them on the baking sheet. Sprinkle with salt and pepper.
5. Bake in the preheated oven for 20 minutes or until lightly browned and al dente. Check the doneness during the baking and remove any well- cooked swoodles.
6. Transfer the swoodles on a large plate and spread with sauce, parsley, and scallions. Toss to serve.

Per Serving

calories: 441 | fat: 33.6g | protein: 12.0g | carbs: 29.6g | fiber: 7.8g | sodium: 479mg

Tomato Sauce and Basil Pesto Fettuccine

Prep time: 15 minutes | Cook time: 15 minutes | Serves 4

4 Roma tomatoes, diced

2 teaspoons no-salt-added tomato paste

1 tablespoon chopped fresh oregano

2 garlic cloves, minced

1 cup low-sodium vegetable soup

½ teaspoon sea salt

1 packed cup fresh basil leaves

¼ cup pine nuts

¼ cup grated Parmesan cheese

2 tablespoons extra-virgin olive oil

1 pound (454 g) cooked whole-grain fettuccine

1. Put the tomatoes, tomato paste, oregano, garlic, vegetable soup, and salt in a skillet. Stir to mix well.
2. Cook over medium heat for 10 minutes or until lightly thickened.
3. Put the remaining ingredients, except for the fettuccine, in a food processor and pulse to combine until smooth.

4. Pour the puréed basil mixture into the tomato mixture, then add the fettuccine. Cook for a few minutes or until heated through and the fettuccine is well coated.

5. Serve immediately.

Per Serving

calories: 389 | fat: 22.7g | protein: 9.7g | carbs: 40.2g | fiber: 4.8g | sodium: 616mg

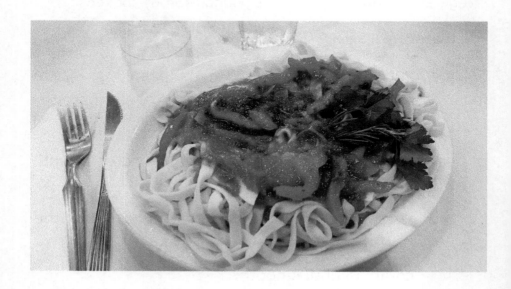

Broccoli and Carrot Pasta Salad

Prep time: 5 minutes | Cook time: 10 minutes | Serves 2

8 ounces (227 g) whole-wheat pasta

2 cups broccoli florets

1 cup peeled and shredded carrots

¼ cup plain Greek yogurt

Juice of 1 lemon

1 teaspoon red pepper flakes

Sea salt and freshly ground pepper, to taste

1. Bring a large pot of lightly salted water to a boil. Add the pasta to the boiling water and cook until al dente, about 8 to 10 minutes. Drain the pasta and let rest for a few minutes.
2. When cooled, combine the pasta with the veggies, yogurt, lemon juice, and red pepper flakes in a large bowl, and stir thoroughly to combine.
3. Taste and season to taste with salt and pepper. Serve immediately.

Per Serving

calories: 428 | fat: 2.9g | protein: 15.9g | carbs: 84.6g | fiber: 11.7g | sodium: 642mg

Bean and Veggie Pasta

Prep time: 10 minutes | Cook time: 15 minutes | Serves 2

16 ounces (454 g) small whole wheat pasta, such as penne, farfalle, or macaroni

5 cups water

1 (15-ounce / 425-g) can cannellini beans, drained and rinsed

1 (14.5-ounce / 411-g) can diced (with juice) or crushed tomatoes

1 yellow onion, chopped

1 red or yellow bell pepper, chopped

2 tablespoons tomato paste

1 tablespoon olive oil

3 garlic cloves, minced

¼ teaspoon crushed red pepper (optional)

1 bunch kale, stemmed and chopped

1 cup sliced basil

½ cup pitted Kalamata olives, chopped

1. Add the pasta, water, beans, tomatoes (with juice if using diced), onion, bell pepper, tomato paste, oil, garlic, and crushed red pepper (if desired), to a large stockpot. Bring to a boil over high heat, stirring often.

2. Reduce the heat to medium-high, add the kale, and cook, continuing to stir often, until the pasta is al dente, about 10 minutes.

3. Remove from the heat and let sit for 5 minutes. Garnish with the basil and olives and serve.

Per Serving

calories: 565 | fat: 17.7g | protein: 18.0g | carbs: 85.5g | fiber: 16.5g | sodium: 540mg

Roasted Ratatouille Pasta

Prep time: 10 minutes | Cook time: 30 minutes | Serves 2

1 small eggplant (about 8 ounces / 227 g)

1 small zucchini

1 portobello mushroom

1 Roma tomato, halved

½ medium sweet red pepper, seeded

½ teaspoon salt, plus additional for the pasta water

1 teaspoon Italian herb seasoning

1 tablespoon olive oil

2 cups farfalle pasta (about 8 ounces / 227 g)

2 tablespoons minced sun-dried tomatoes in olive oil with herbs

2 tablespoons prepared pesto

1. Slice the ends off the eggplant and zucchini. Cut them lengthwise into ½- inch slices.
2. Place the eggplant, zucchini, mushroom, tomato, and red pepper in a large bowl and sprinkle with ½ teaspoon of salt. Using your hands, toss the vegetables well so that they're covered evenly with the salt. Let them rest for about 10 minutes.

3. While the vegetables are resting, preheat the oven to 400°F (205°C). Line a baking sheet with parchment paper.

4. When the oven is hot, drain off any liquid from the vegetables and pat them dry with a paper towel. Add the Italian herb seasoning and olive oil to the vegetables and toss well to coat both sides.

5. Lay the vegetables out in a single layer on the baking sheet. Roast them for 15 to 20 minutes, flipping them over after about 10 minutes or once they start to brown on the underside. When the vegetables are charred in spots, remove them from the oven.

6. While the vegetables are roasting, fill a large saucepan with water. Add salt and cook the pasta until al dente, about 8 to 10 minutes. Drain the pasta, reserving ½ cup of the pasta water.

7. When cool enough to handle, cut the vegetables into large chunks (about 2 inches) and add them to the hot pasta.

8. Stir in the sun-dried tomatoes and pesto and toss everything well. Serve immediately.

Per Serving

calories: 613 | fat: 16.0g | protein: 23.1g | carbs: 108.5g | fiber: 23.0g | sodium: 775mg

Lentil and Mushroom Pasta

Prep time: 10 minutes | Cook time: 50 minutes | Serves 2

2 tablespoons olive oil

1 large yellow onion, finely diced

2 portobello mushrooms, trimmed and chopped finely

2 tablespoons tomato paste

3 garlic cloves, chopped

1 teaspoon oregano

2½ cups water

1 cup brown lentils

1 (28-ounce / 794-g) can diced tomatoes with basil (with juice if diced)

1 tablespoon balsamic vinegar

Salt and black pepper, to taste

Chopped basil, for garnish

8 ounces (227 g) pasta of choice, cooked

1. Place a large stockpot over medium heat and add the olive oil. Once the oil is hot, add the onion and mushrooms. Cover and cook until both are soft, about 5 minutes. Add the tomato paste, garlic, and oregano and cook 2 minutes, stirring constantly.

2. Stir in the water and lentils. Bring to a boil, then reduce the heat to medium-low and cook covered for 5 minutes.
3. Add the tomatoes (and juice if using diced) and vinegar. Reduce the heat to low and cook until the lentils are tender, about 30 minutes.
4. Remove from the heat and season with salt and pepper to taste. Garnish with the basil and serve over the cooked pasta.

Per Serving

calories: 463 | fat: 15.9g | protein: 12.5g | carbs: 70.8g | fiber: 16.9g | sodium: 155mg

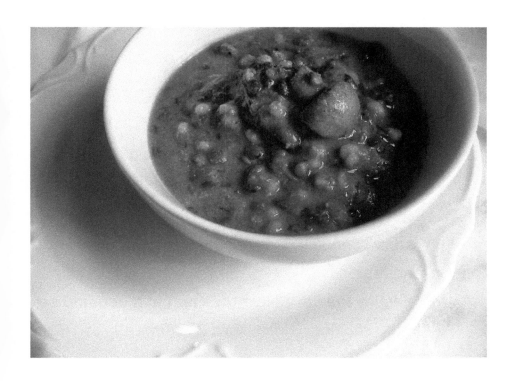

Tomato Basil Pasta

Prep time: 3 minutes | Cook time: 2 minutes | Serves 2

2 cups dried campanelle or similar pasta

1¾ cups vegetable stock

½ teaspoon salt, plus more as needed

2 tomatoes, cut into large dices

1 or 2 pinches red pepper flakes

½ teaspoon garlic powder

½ teaspoon dried oregano

10 to 12 fresh sweet basil leaves

Freshly ground black pepper, to taste

1. In your Instant Pot, stir together the pasta, stock, and salt. Scatter the tomatoes on top (do not stir).

2. Secure the lid. Select the Manual mode and set the cooking time for 2 minutes at High Pressure.

3. Once cooking is complete, do a quick pressure release. Carefully open the lid.

4. Stir in the red pepper flakes, oregano, and garlic powder. If there's more than a few tablespoons of liquid in the bottom, select

Sauté and cook for 2 to 3 minutes until it evaporates.

5. When ready to serve, chiffonade the basil and stir it in. Taste and season with more salt and pepper, as needed. Serve warm.

Per Serving

calories: 415 | fat: 2.0g | protein: 15.2g | carbs: 84.2g | fiber: 5.0g | sodium: 485mg

Lentil Risotto

Prep time: 10 minutes | Cook time: 20 minutes | Serves 2

½ tablespoon olive oil

½ medium onion, chopped

½ cup dry lentils, soaked overnight

½ celery stalk, chopped

1 sprig parsley, chopped

½ cup Arborio (short-grain Italian) rice

1 garlic clove, lightly mashed

2 cups vegetable stock

1. Press the Sauté button to heat your Instant Pot.
2. Add the oil and onion to the Instant Pot and sauté for 5 minutes.
3. Add the remaining ingredients to the Instant Pot, stirring well.
4. Secure the lid. Select the Manual mode and set the cooking time for 15 minutes at High Pressure.
5. Once cooking is complete, do a natural pressure release for 20 minutes, then release any remaining pressure. Carefully open the lid.
6. Stir and serve hot.

Per Serving

calories: 261 | fat: 3.6g | protein: 10.6g | carbs: 47.1g | fiber: 8.4g | sodium: 247mg

Bulgur Pilaf with Kale and Tomatoes

Prep time: 10 minutes | Cook time: 10 minutes | Serves 2

2 tablespoons olive oilzxcvn,

2 cloves garlic, minced

1 bunch kale, trimmed and cut into bite-sized pieces

Juice of 1 lemon

2 cups cooked bulgur wheat

1 pint cherry tomatoes, halved

Sea salt and freshly ground pepper, to taste

1. Heat the olive oil in a large skillet over medium heat. Add the garlic and sauté for 1 minute.
2. Add the kale leaves and stir to coat. Cook for 5 minutes until leaves are cooked through and thoroughly wilted.
3. Add the lemon juice, bulgur and tomatoes. Season with sea salt and freshly ground pepper to taste, then serve.

Per Serving

calories: 300 | fat: 14.0g | protein: 6.2g | carbs: 37.8g | fiber: 8.7g | sodium: 595mg

Cranberry and Almond Quinoa

Prep time: 5 minutes | Cook time: 10 minutes | Serves 2

2 cups water

1 cup quinoa, rinsed

¼ cup salted sunflower seeds

½ cup slivered almonds

1 cup dried cranberries

1. Combine water and quinoa in the Instant Pot.
2. Secure the lid. Select the Manual mode and set the cooking time for 10 minutes at High Pressure.
3. Once cooking is complete, do a quick pressure release. Carefully open the lid.
4. Add sunflower seeds, almonds, and dried cranberries and gently mix until well combined.
5. Serve hot.

Per Serving

calories: 445 | fat: 14.8g | protein: 15.1g | carbs: 64.1g | fiber: 10.2g | sodium: 113mg

Pork and Spinach Spaghetti

Prep time: 15 minutes | Cook time: 16 minutes | Serves 4

2 tablespoons olive oil

½ cup onion, chopped

1 garlic clove, minced

1 pound (454 g) ground pork

2 cups water

1 (14-ounce / 397-g) can diced tomatoes, drained

½ cup sun-dried tomatoes

1 tablespoon dried oregano

1 teaspoon Italian seasoning

1 fresh jalapeño chile, stemmed, seeded, and minced

1 teaspoon salt

8 ounces (227 g) dried spaghetti, halved

1 cup spinach

1. Warm oil onSauté. Add onion and garlic and cook for 2 minutes until softened. Stir in pork and cook for 5 minutes. Stir in jalapeño, water, sun- dried tomatoes, Italian seasoning, oregano, diced tomatoes, and salt with the chicken; mix spaghetti and press to submerge into the sauce.

2. Seal the lid and cook on High Pressure for 9 minutes. Release the pressure quickly. Stir in

spinach, close lid again, and simmer on Keep Warm for 5 minutes until spinach is wilted.

Per Serving

calories: 621 | fat: 32.2g | protein: 29.1g | carbs: 53.9g | fiber: 5.9g | sodium: 738mg

Gouda Beef and Spinach Fettuccine

Prep time: 10 minutes | Cook time: 15 minutes | Serves 6

10 ounces (283 g) ground beef

1 pound (454 g) fettuccine pasta

1 cup gouda cheese, shredded

1 cup fresh spinach, torn

1 medium onion, chopped

2 cups tomatoes, diced

1 tablespoon olive oil

1 teaspoon salt

½ teaspoon ground black pepper

1. Heat the olive oil on Sauté mode in the Instant Pot. Stir-fry the beef and onion for 5 minutes. Add the pasta. Pour water enough to cover and season with salt and pepper. Cook on High Pressure for 5 minutes.
2. Do a quick release. Press Sauté and stir in the tomato and spinach; cook for 5 minutes. Top with Gouda to serve.

Per Serving

calories: 493 | fat: 17.7g | protein: 20.6g | carbs: 64.3g | fiber: 9.5g | sodium: 561mg

Rigatoni and Zucchini Minestrone

Prep time: 20 minutes | Cook time: 7 minutes | Serves 4

3 tablespoons olive oil

1 onion, diced

1 celery stalk, diced

1 large carrot, peeled and diced

14 ounces (397 g) canned chopped tomatoes

4 ounces (113 g) rigatoni

3 cups water

1 cup chopped zucchini

1 bay leaf

1 teaspoon mixed herbs

¼ teaspoon cayenne pepper

½ teaspoon salt

¼ cup shredded Pecorino Romano cheese

1 garlic clove, minced

1 ⬚ cup olive oil-based pesto

1. Heat oil on Sauté and cook onion, celery, garlic, and carrot for 3 minutes, stirring occasionally until the vegetables are softened. Stir in rigatoni, tomatoes, water, zucchini, bay leaf, herbs, cayenne, and salt.

2. Seal the lid and cook on High for 4 minutes. Do a natural pressure release for 5 minutes. Adjust

the taste of the soup with salt and black pepper, and remove the bay leaf.

3. Ladle the soup into serving bowls and drizzle the pesto over. Serve with the garlic toasts.

Per Serving

calories: 278 | fat: 23.4g | protein: 6.7g | carbs: 12.2g | fiber: 3.5g | sodium: 793mg

Asparagus and Broccoli Primavera Farfalle

Prep time: 15 minutes | Cook time: 12 minutes | Serves 4

1 bunch asparagus, trimmed, cut into 1-inch pieces

2 cups broccoli florets

3 tablespoons olive oil

3 teaspoons salt

10 ounces (283 g) egg noodles

3 garlic cloves, minced

2½ cups vegetable stock

½ cup heavy cream

1 cup small tomatoes, halved

¼ cup chopped basil

½ cup grated Parmesan cheese

1. Pour 2 cups of water, add the noodles, 2 tablespoons of olive oil, garlic and salt. Place a trivet over the water. Combine asparagus, broccoli, remaining olive oil and salt in a bowl. Place the vegetables on the trivet.
2. Seal the lid and cook on Steam for 12 minutes on High. Do a quick release. Remove the

vegetables to a plate. Stir the heavy cream and tomatoes in the pasta. Press Sauté and simmer the cream until desired consistency. Gently mix in the asparagus and broccoli. Garnish with basil and Parmesan, to serve.

Per Serving

calories: 544 | fat: 23.8g | protein: 18.5g | carbs: 66.1g | fiber: 6.0g | sodium: 2354mg

Super Cheesy Tagliatelle

Prep time: 10 minutes | Cook time: 20 minutes | Serves 6

¼ cup goat cheese, chevre

¼ cup grated Pecorino cheese

½ cup grated Parmesan

1 cup heavy cream

½ cup grated Gouda

2 tablespoons olive oil

1 tablespoon Italian Seasoning mix

1 cup vegetable broth

1 pound (454 g) tagliatelle

1. In a bowl, mix goat cheese, pecorino, Parmesan, and heavy cream. Stir in Italian seasoning. Transfer to your instant pot. Stir in the broth and olive oil.
2. Seal the lid and cook on High Pressure for 4 minutes. Do a quick release.
1. Meanwhile, drop the tagliatelle in boiling water and cook for 6 minutes.
2. Remove the instant pot's lid and stir in the tagliatelle. Top with grated gouda and let simmer for about 10 minutes on Sauté mode.

Per Serving

calories: 511 | fat: 22.0g | protein: 14.5g | carbs: 65.7g | fiber: 9.0g | sodium: 548mg

Chickpea Curry

Prep time: 10 minutes | Cook time: 24 minutes | Serves 4

½ cup raw chickpeas

1½ tablespoons cooking oil

½ cup chopped onions

1 bay leaf

½ tablespoon grated garlic

¼ tablespoon grated ginger

¾ cup water

1 cup fresh tomato purée

½ green chili, finely chopped

¼ teaspoon turmeric

½ teaspoon coriander powder

1 teaspoon chili powder

1 cup chopped baby spinach

Salt, to taste

Boiled white rice, for serving

1. Add the oil and onions to the Instant Pot. Sauté for 5 minutes.
2. Stir in ginger, garlic paste, green chili and bay leaf. Cook for 1 minute, then add all the spices.
3. Add the chickpeas, tomato purée and the water to the pot.
4. Cover and secure the lid. Turn its pressure release handle to the sealing position.

5. Cook on the Manual function with High Pressure for 15 minutes.

6. After the beep, do a Natural release for 20 minutes.

7. Stir in spinach and cook for 3 minutes on the Sauté setting.

8. Serve hot with boiled white rice.

Per Serving

calories: 176 | fat: 6.8g | protein: 6.7g | carbs: 24.1g | fiber: 5.1g | sodium: 185mg

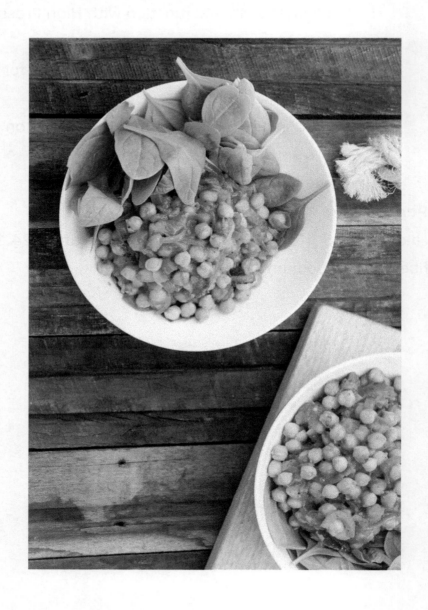

Sides, Salads, and Soups

Greek Salad with Dressing

Prep time: 10 minutes | Cook time: 0 minutes | Serves 4 to 6

1 head iceberg lettuce

2 cups cherry tomatoes

1 large cucumber

1 medium onion

¼ cup lemon juice

½ cup extra-virgin olive oil

1 teaspoon salt

1 clove garlic, minced

1 cup Kalamata olives, pitted

1 (6-ounce / 170-g) package feta cheese, crumbled

1. Cut the lettuce into 1-inch pieces and put them in a large salad bowl.
2. Cut the tomatoes in half and add them to the salad bowl.
3. Slice the cucumber into bite-sized pieces and add them to the salad bowl.
4. Thinly slice the onion and add it to the salad bowl.

5. In a separate bowl, whisk together the olive oil, lemon juice, salt, and garlic. Pour the dressing over the salad and gently toss to evenly coat.

6. Top the salad with the Kalamata olives and feta cheese and serve.

Per Serving

calories: 539 | fat: 50.0g | protein: 9.0g | carbs: 18.0g | fiber: 4.0g | sodium: 1758mg

Tricolor Summer Salad

Prep time: 10 minutes | Cook time: 0 minutes | Serves 3 to 4

¼ cup while balsamic vinegar

2 tablespoons Dijon mustard

1 tablespoon sugar

½ teaspoon garlic salt

½ teaspoon freshly ground black pepper

¼ cup extra-virgin olive oil

1½ cups chopped orange, yellow, and red tomatoes

½ cucumber, peeled and diced

1 small red onion, thinly sliced

¼ cup crumbled feta (optional)

1. In a small bowl, whisk the vinegar, mustard, sugar, pepper, and garlic salt. Then slowly whisk in the olive oil.
2. In a large bowl, add the tomatoes, cucumber, and red onion. Add the dressing. Toss once or twice, and serve with the feta crumbles (if desired) sprinkled on top.

Per Serving

calories: 246 | fat: 18.0g | protein: 1.0g | carbs: 19.0g | fiber: 2.0g | sodium: 483mg

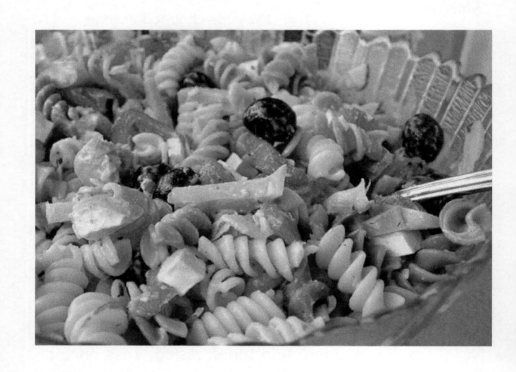

Chicken and Pastina Soup

Prep time: 5 minutes | Cook time: 20 minutes | Serves 6

1 tablespoon extra-virgin olive oil

2 garlic cloves, minced

3 cups packed chopped kale; center ribs removed

1 cup minced carrots

8 cups no-salt-added chicken or vegetable broth

¼ teaspoon kosher or sea salt

¼ teaspoon freshly ground black pepper

¾ cup uncooked acini de pepe or pastina pasta

2 cups shredded cooked chicken (about 12 ounces / 340 g)

3 tablespoons grated Parmesan cheese

1. In a large stockpot over medium heat, heat the oil. Add the garlic and cook for 30 seconds, stirring frequently. Add the kale and carrots and cook for 5 minutes, stirring occasionally.

2. Add the broth, salt, and pepper, and turn the heat to high. Bring the broth to a boil, and add the pasta. Reduce the heat to medium and cook for 10 minutes, or until the pasta is cooked

through, stirring every few minutes so the pasta doesn't stick to the bottom. Add the chicken, and cook for another 2 minutes to warm through.

3. Ladle the soup into six bowls. Top each with ½ tablespoon of cheese and serve.

Per Serving

calories: 275 | fat: 19.0g | protein: 16.0g | carbs: 11.0g | fiber: 2.0g | sodium: 298mg

Green Bean and Halloumi Salad

Prep time: 20 minutes | Cook time: 5 minutes | Serves 2

Dressing:

¼ cup unsweetened coconut milk

1 tablespoon olive oil

2 teaspoons freshly squeezed lemon juice

¼ teaspoon garlic powder

¼ teaspoon onion powder Pinch salt

Pinch freshly ground black pepper

Salad:

½ pound (227 g) fresh green beans, trimmed

2 ounces (57 g) Halloumi cheese, sliced into 2 (½-inch-thick) slices

½ cup halved cherry or grape tomatoes

¼ cup thinly sliced sweet onion

Make the Dressing

1. Combine the coconut milk, olive oil, lemon juice, onion powder, garlic powder, salt, and pepper in a small bowl and whisk well. Set aside.

Make the Salad

2. Fill a medium-size pot with about 1 inch of water and add the green beans. Cover and steam them for about 3 to 4 minutes, or just until beans are tender. Do not overcook. Drain beans, rinse them immediately with cold water, and set them aside to cool.

3. Heat a nonstick skillet over medium-high heat and place the slices of Halloumi in the hot pan. After about 2 minutes, check to see if the cheese is golden on the bottom. If it is, flip the slices and cook for another minute or until the second side is golden.

4. Remove cheese from the pan and cut each piece into cubes (about 1-inch square).

5. Place the green beans, halloumi slices, tomatoes, and onion in a large bowl and toss to combine.

6. Drizzle the dressing over the salad and toss well to combine. Serve immediately.

Per Serving

calories: 274 | fat: 18.1g | protein: 8.0g | carbs: 16.8g | fiber: 5.1g | sodium: 499mg

Citrus Salad with Kale and Fennel

Prep time: 15 minutes | Cook time: 0 minutes | Serves 2

Dressing:

3 tablespoons olive oil

2 tablespoons fresh orange juice

1 tablespoon blood orange vinegar, other orange vinegar, or cider vinegar

1 tablespoon honey

Salt and freshly ground black pepper, to taste

Salad:

2 cups packed baby kale

1 medium navel or blood orange, segmented

½ small fennel bulb, stems and leaves removed, sliced into matchsticks

3 tablespoons toasted pecans, chopped

2 ounces (57 g) goat cheese, crumbled

Make the Dressing

1. Mix the olive oil, orange juice, vinegar, and honey in a small bowl and whisk to combine. Season with salt and pepper to taste. Set aside.

Make the Salad

2. Divide the baby kale, orange segments, fennel, pecans, and goat cheese evenly between two plates.

3. Drizzle half of the dressing over each salad and serve.

Per Serving

calories: 503 | fat: 39.1g | protein: 13.2g | carbs: 31.2g | fiber: 6.1g | sodium: 156mg

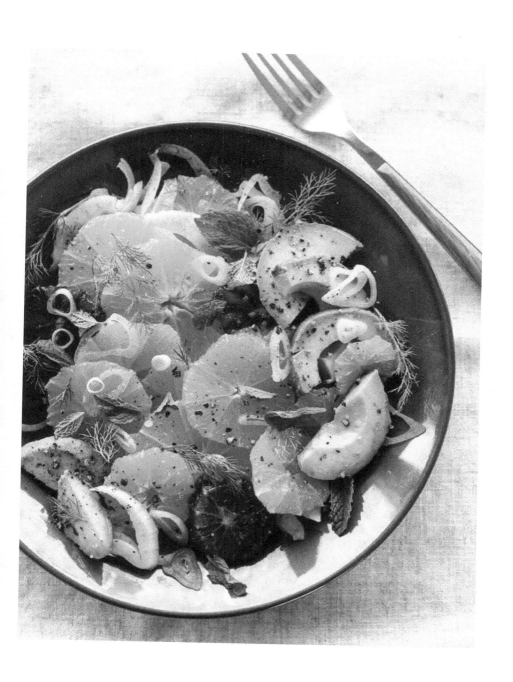

Arugula, Watermelon, and Feta Salad

Prep time: 10 minutes | Cook time: 0 minutes | Serves 2

3 cups packed arugula

2½ cups watermelon, cut into bite-size cubes

2 ounces (57 g) feta cheese, crumbled

2 tablespoons balsamic glaze

1. Divide the arugula between two plates.
2. Divide the watermelon cubes between the beds of arugula.
3. Scatter half of the feta cheese over each salad.
4. Drizzle about 1 tablespoon of the glaze (or more if desired) over each salad. Serve immediately.

Per Serving

calories: 157 | fat: 6.9g | protein: 6.1g | carbs: 22.0g | fiber: 1.1g | sodium: 328mg

Mediterranean Tomato Hummus Soup

Prep time: 10 minutes | Cook time: 10 minutes | Serves 2

1 (14.5-ounce / 411-g) can crushed tomatoes with basil

2 cups low-sodium chicken stock

1 cup roasted red pepper hummus

Salt, to taste

¼ cup thinly sliced fresh basil leaves, for garnish (optional)

1. Combine the canned tomatoes, hummus, and chicken stock in a blender and blend until smooth. Pour the mixture into a saucepan and bring it to a boil. Season with salt to taste.
2. Serve garnished with the fresh basil, if desired.

Per Serving

calories: 147 | fat: 6.2g | protein: 5.2g | carbs: 20.1g | fiber: 4.1g | sodium: 682mg

Vegetable Fagioli Soup

Prep time: 30 minutes | Cook time: 60 minutes | Serves 2

1 tablespoon olive oil

2 medium carrots, diced

2 medium celery stalks, diced

½ medium onion, diced

1 large garlic clove, minced

3 tablespoons tomato paste

4 cups low-sodium vegetable broth

1 cup packed kale, stemmed and chopped

1 (15-ounce / 425-g) can red kidney beans, drained and rinsed

1 (15-ounce / 425-g) can cannellini beans, drained and rinsed

½ cup chopped fresh basil

Salt and freshly ground black pepper, to taste

1. Heat the olive oil in a stockpot over medium-high heat. Add the carrots, celery, onion, and garlic and sauté for 10 minutes, or until the vegetables start to turn golden.

2. Stir in the tomato paste and cook for about 30 seconds.

3. Add the vegetable broth and bring the soup to a boil. Cover and reduce the heat to low. Cook the soup for 45 minutes, or until the carrots are tender.

4. Using an immersion blender, purée the soup so that it's partly smooth, but with some chunks of vegetables.

5. Add the kale, beans, and basil. Season with salt and pepper to taste, then serve.

Per Serving

calories: 217 | fat: 4.2g | protein: 10.0g | carbs: 36.2g | fiber: 10.2g | sodium: 482mg

Avgolemono (Lemon Chicken Soup)

Prep time: 15 minutes | Cook time: 60 minutes | Serves 2

½ large onion

2 medium carrots

1 celery stalk

1 garlic clove

5 cups low-sodium chicken stock

¼ cup brown rice

1½ cups (about 5 ounces / 142 g) shredded rotisserie chicken

3 tablespoons freshly squeezed lemon juice

1 egg yolk

2 tablespoons chopped fresh dill

2 tablespoons chopped fresh parsley

Salt, to taste

1. Put the onion, carrots, celery, and garlic in a food processor and pulse until the vegetables are minced.
2. Add the vegetables and chicken stock to a stockpot and bring it to a boil over high heat.
3. Reduce the heat to medium-low and add the rice, shredded chicken and lemon juice. Cover

and let the soup simmer for 40 minutes, or until the rice is cooked.

4. In a small bowl, whisk the egg yolk lightly. Slowly, while whisking with one hand, pour about ½ of a ladle of the broth into the egg yolk to warm, or temper, the yolk. Slowly add another ladle of broth and continue to whisk.

5. Remove the soup from the heat and pour the whisked egg yolk–broth mixture into the pot. Stir well to combine.

6. Add the fresh dill and parsley. Season with salt to taste and serve.

Per Serving

calories: 172 | fat: 4.2g | protein: 18.2g | carbs: 16.1g | fiber: 2.1g | sodium: 232mg

Vegetable Mains

Cabbage Stuffed Acorn Squash

Prep time: 15 minutes | Cook time: 23 minutes | Serves 4

½ tablespoon olive oil

2 medium Acorn squashes

¼ small yellow onion, chopped

1 jalapeño pepper, chopped

½ cup green onions, chopped

½ cup carrots, chopped

¼ cup cabbage, chopped

1 garlic clove, minced

½ (6-ounce / 170-g) can sugar-free tomato sauce

½ tablespoon chili powder

½ tablespoon ground cumin

Salt and freshly ground black pepper to taste

2 cups water

¼ cup Cheddar cheese, shredded

1. Pour the water into the instant pot and place the trivet inside.

64

2. Slice the squash into 2 halves and remove the seeds.
3. Place over the trivet, skin side down, and sprinkle some salt and pepper over it.
4. Secure the lid and cook on Manual for 15 minutes at High Pressure.
5. Release the pressure naturally and remove the lid. Empty the pot into a bowl.
6. Now add the oil, onion, and garlic in the instant pot and Sauté for 5 minutes.
7. Stir in the remaining vegetables and stir-fry for 3 minutes.
8. Add the remaining ingredients and secure the lid.
9. Cook on Manual function for 2 minutes at High Pressure.
10. After the beep, natural release the pressure and remove the lid.
11. Stuff the squashes with the prepared mixture and serve warm.

Per Serving

calories: 163 | fat: 5.1g | protein: 4.8g | carbs: 28.4g | fiber: 4.9g | sodium: 146mg

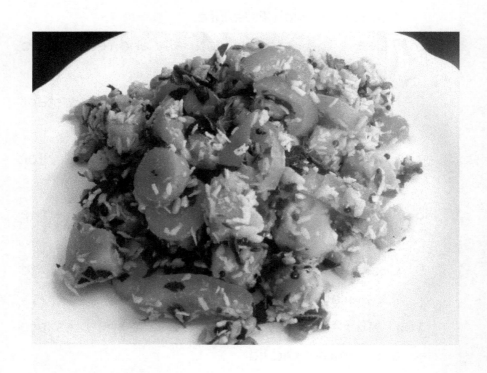

Creamy Potato Curry

Prep time: 10 minutes | Cook time: 18 minutes | Serves 4

¾ large yellow or white onion, chopped

1½ ribs celery, chopped

¼ cup carrots, diced

¼ cup green onions

½ cup coconut milk

¾ tablespoon garlic, chopped

1½ cups water

1 pound (454 g) white potatoes, peeled and diced

¼ cup heavy cream

¼ teaspoon thyme

¼ teaspoon rosemary

½ tablespoon black pepper

¾ cup peas Salt, to taste

2 tablespoons fresh cilantro for garnishing, chopped

1. Add the oil and all the vegetables in the instant pot and Sauté for 5 minutes.
2. Stir in the remaining ingredients and secure the lid.
3. Cook on Manual function for 13 minutes at High Pressure.

4. Once it beeps, natural release the pressure and remove the lid.

5. Garnish with fresh cilantro and serve hot.

Per Serving

calories: 210 | fat: 10.1g | protein: 4.1g | carbs: 27.6g | fiber: 4.7g | sodium: 74mg

Mushroom and Spinach Stuffed Peppers

Prep time: 15 minutes | Cook time: 8 minutes | Serves 7

7 mini sweet peppers

1 cup button mushrooms, minced

5 ounces (142 g) organic baby spinach

½ teaspoon fresh garlic

½ teaspoon coarse sea salt

¼ teaspoon cracked mixed pepper

2 tablespoons water

1 tablespoon olive oil

Organic Mozzarella cheese, diced

1. Put the sweet peppers and water in the instant pot and Sauté for 2 minutes.
2. Remove the peppers and put the olive oil into the pot.
3. Stir in the mushrooms, garlic, spices and spinach.
4. Cook on Sauté until the mixture is dry.
5. Stuff each sweet pepper with the cheese and spinach mixture.

6. Bake the stuffed peppers in an oven for 6 minutes at 400ºF (205ºC).

7. Once done, serve hot.

Per Serving

calories: 81 | fat: 2.4g | protein: 4.1g | carbs: 13.2g | fiber: 2.4g | sodium: 217mg

Black Bean and Corn Tortilla Bowls

Prep time: 10 minutes | Cook time: 8 minutes | Serves 4

1½ cups vegetable broth

½ cup tomatoes, undrained diced

1 small onion, diced

2 garlic cloves, finely minced

1 teaspoon chili powder

1 teaspoon cumin

½ teaspoon paprika

½ teaspoon ground coriander

Salt and pepper to taste

½ cup carrots, diced

2 small potatoes, cubed

½ cup bell pepper, chopped

½ can black beans, drained and rinsed

1 cup frozen corn kernels

½ tablespoon lime juice

2 tablespoons cilantro for topping, chopped

Whole-wheat tortilla chips

1. Add the oil and all the vegetables into the instant pot and Sauté for 3 minutes.

71

2. Add all the spices, corn, lime juice, and broth, along with the beans, to the pot.

3. Seal the lid and cook on Manual setting at High Pressure for 5 minutes.

4. Once done, natural release the pressure when the timer goes off. Remove the lid.

5. To serve, put the prepared mixture into a bowl.

6. Top with tortilla chips and fresh cilantro.

7. Serve.

Per Serving

calories: 183 | fat: 0.9g | protein: 7.1g | carbs: 39.8g | fiber: 8.3g | sodium: 387mg

Cauliflower and Broccoli Bowls

Prep time: 5 minutes | Cook time: 7 minutes | Serves 3

½ medium onion, diced

2 teaspoons olive oil

1 garlic clove, minced

½ cup tomato paste

½ pound (227 g) frozen cauliflower

½ pound (227 g) broccoli florets

½ cup vegetable broth

½ teaspoon paprika

¼ teaspoon dried thyme

2 pinches sea salt

1. Add the oil, onion and garlic into the instant pot and Sauté for 2 minutes.
2. Add the broth, tomato paste, cauliflower, broccoli, and all the spices, to the pot.
3. Secure the lid. Cook on the Manual setting at with pressure for 5 minutes.
4. After the beep, Quick release the pressure and remove the lid.
5. Stir well and serve hot.

Per Serving

calories: 109 | fat: 3.8g | protein: 6.1g | carbs: 16.7g | fiber: 6.1g | sodium: 265mg

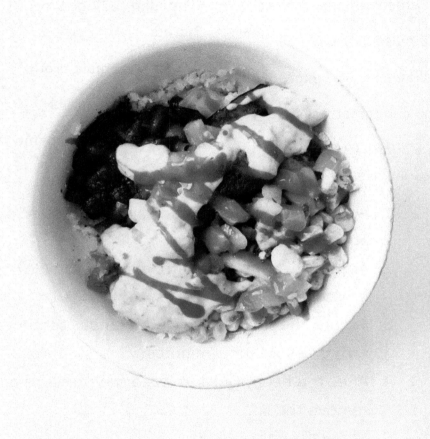

Radish and Cabbage Congee

Prep time: 5 minutes | Cook time: 20 minutes | Serves 3

1 cup carrots, diced

½ cup radish, diced

6 cups vegetable broth

Salt, to taste

1½ cups short grain rice, rinsed

1 tablespoon grated fresh ginger

4 cups cabbage, shredded

Green onions for garnishing, chopped

1. Add all the ingredients, except the cabbage and green onions, into the instant pot.
2. Select the Porridge function and cook on the default time and settings.
3. After the beep, Quick release the pressure and remove the lid
4. Stir in the shredded cabbage and cover with the lid.
5. Serve after 10 minutes with chopped green onions on top.

Per Serving

calories: 438 | fat: 0.8g | protein: 8.7g | carbs: 98.4g | fiber: 6.7g | sodium: 1218mg

Potato and Broccoli Medley

Prep time: 10 minutes | Cook time: 20 minutes | Serves 3

1 tablespoon olive oil

½ white onion, diced

1½ cloves garlic, finely chopped

1 pound (454 g) potatoes, cut into chunks

1 pound (454 g) broccoli florets, diced

1 pound (454 g) baby carrots, cut in half

¼ cup vegetable broth

½ teaspoon Italian seasoning

½ teaspoon Spike original seasoning

Fresh parsley for garnishing

1. Put the oil and onion into the instant pot and Sauté for 5 minutes.
2. Stir in the carrots, and garlic and stir-fry for 5 minutes.
3. Add the remaining ingredients and secure the lid.
4. Cook on the Manual function for 10 minutes at High Pressure.
5. After the beep, Quick release the pressure and remove the lid.

6. Stir gently and garnish with fresh parsley , then serve.

Per Serving

calories: 256 | fat: 5.6g | protein: 9.1g | carbs: 46.1g | fiber: 12.2g | sodium: 274mg

Mushroom and Potato Oat Burgers

Prep time: 20 minutes | Cook time: 21 minutes | Serves 5

½ cup minced onion

1 teaspoon grated fresh ginger

½ cup minced mushrooms

½ cup red lentils, rinsed

¾ sweet potato, peeled and diced

1 cup vegetable stock

2 tablespoons hemp seeds

2 tablespoons chopped parsley

2 tablespoons chopped cilantro

1 tablespoon curry powder

1 cup quick oats

Brown rice flour, optional

5 tomato slices

Lettuce leaves

5 whole-wheat buns

1. Add the oil, ginger, mushrooms and onion into the instant pot and Sauté for 5 minutes.
2. Stir in the lentils, stock, and the sweet potatoes.
3. Secure the lid and cook on the Manual function for 6 minutes at High Pressure.

4. After the beep, natural release the pressure and remove the lid.

5. Meanwhile, heat the oven to 375ºF (190ºC) and line a baking tray with parchment paper.

6. Mash the prepared lentil mixture with a potato masher.

7. Add the oats and the remaining spices. Put in some brown rice flour if the mixture is not thick enough.

8. Wet your hands and prepare 5 patties, using the mixture, and place them on the baking tray.

9. Bake the patties for 10 minutes in the preheated oven.

10. Slice the buns in half and stack each with a tomato slice, a vegetable patty and lettuce leaves.

11. Serve and enjoy.

Per Serving

calories: 266 | fat: 5.3g | protein: 14.5g | carbs: 48.7g | fiber: 9.6g | sodium: 276mg

Potato, Corn, and Spinach Medley

Prep time: 10 minutes | Cook time: 10 minutes | Serves 6

1 tablespoon olive oil

3 scallions, chopped

½ cup onion, chopped

2 large white potatoes, peeled and diced

1 tablespoon ginger, grated

3 cups frozen corn kernels

1 cup vegetable stock

1 tablespoon fish sauce

2 tablespoons light soy sauce

2 large cloves garlic, diced

1 teaspoon white pepper

1 teaspoon salt

3-4 handfuls baby spinach leaves

Juice of ½ lemon

1. Put the oil, ginger, garlic and onions in the instant pot and Sauté for 5 minutes.
2. Add all the remaining ingredients except the spinach leaves and lime juice
3. Secure the lid and cook on the Manual setting for 5 minutes at High Pressure.
4. After the beep, Quick release the pressure and remove the lid.

5. Add the spinach and cook for 3 minutes on Sauté

6. Drizzle the lime juice over the dish and serve hot.

Per Serving

calories: 217 | fat: 3.4g | protein: 6.5g | carbs: 44.5g | fiber: 6.3g | sodium: 892mg

Italian Zucchini Pomodoro

Prep time: 10 minutes | Cook time: 12 minutes | Serves 4

1 tablespoon avocado oil

1 large onion, peeled and diced

3 cloves garlic, minced

1 (28-ounce / 794-g) can diced tomatoes, including juice

½ cup water

1 tablespoon Italian seasoning

1 teaspoon sea salt

½ teaspoon ground black pepper

2 medium zucchini, spiraled

1. Press Sauté button on the Instant Pot. Heat avocado oil. Add onions and stir-fry for 3 to 5 minutes until translucent. Add garlic and cook for an additional minute. Add tomatoes, water, Italian seasoning, salt, and pepper. Add zucchini and toss to combine. Lock lid.

2. Press the Manual button and adjust time to 1 minute. When timer beeps, let pressure release naturally for 5 minutes. Quick release any additional pressure until float valve drops and then unlock lid.

3. Transfer zucchini to four bowls. Press Sauté button, press Adjust button to change the temperature to Less, and simmer sauce in the Instant Pot unlidded for 5 minutes. Ladle over zucchini and serve immediately.

Per Serving

calories: 92 | fat: 4.1g | protein: 2.5g | carbs: 13.1g | fiber: 5.1g | sodium: 980mg

Mushroom Swoodles

Prep time: 5 minutes | Cook time: 3 minutes | Serves 4

2 tablespoons coconut aminos

1 tablespoon white vinegar

2 teaspoons olive oil

1 teaspoon sesame oil

1 tablespoon honey

¼ teaspoon red pepper flakes

3 cloves garlic, minced

1 large sweet potato, peeled and spiraled

1 pound (454 g) shiitake mushrooms, sliced

1 cup vegetable broth

¼ cup chopped fresh parsley

1. In a large bowl, whisk together coconut aminos, vinegar, olive oil, sesame oil, honey, red pepper flakes, and garlic.
2. Toss sweet potato and shiitake mushrooms in sauce. Refrigerate covered for 30 minutes.
3. Pour vegetable broth into Instant Pot. Add trivet. Lower steamer basket onto trivet and add the sweet potato mixture to the basket. Lock lid.
4. Press the Manual button and adjust time to 3 minutes. When timer beeps, let pressure

release naturally for 5 minutes. Quick release any additional pressure until float valve drops and then unlock lid.

5. Remove basket from the Instant Pot and distribute sweet potatoes and mushrooms evenly among four bowls; pour liquid from the Instant Pot over bowls and garnish with chopped parsley.

Per Serving

calories: 127 | fat: 4.0g | protein: 4.2g | carbs: 20.9g | fiber: 4.1g | sodium: 671mg

Rice, Corn, and Bean Stuffed Peppers

Prep time: 15 minutes | Cook time: 15 minutes | Serves 4

4 large bell peppers

2 cups cooked white rice

1 medium onion, peeled and diced

3 small Roma tomatoes, diced

¼ cup marinara sauce

1 cup corn kernels (cut from the cob is preferred)

¼ cup sliced black olives

¼ cup canned cannellini beans, rinsed and drained

¼ cup canned black beans, rinsed and drained

1 teaspoon sea salt

1 teaspoon garlic powder

½ cup vegetable broth

2 tablespoons grated Parmesan cheese

1. Cut off the bell pepper tops as close to the tops as possible. Hollow out and discard seeds. Poke a few small holes in the bottom of the peppers to allow drippings to drain.
2. In a medium bowl, combine remaining ingredients except for broth and Parmesan

cheese. Stuff equal amounts of mixture into each of the bell peppers.

3. Place trivet into the Instant Pot and pour in the broth. Set the peppers upright on the trivet. Lock lid.

4. Press the Manual button and adjust time to 15 minutes. When timer beeps, let pressure release naturally until float valve drops and then unlock lid.

5. Serve immediately and garnish with Parmesan cheese.

Per Serving

calories: 265 | fat: 3.0g | protein: 8.1g | carbs: 53.1g | fiber: 8.0g | sodium: 834mg

Carrot and Turnip Purée

Prep time: 10 minutes | Cook time: 10 minutes | Serves 6

2 tablespoons olive oil, divided

3 large turnips, peeled and quartered

4 large carrots, peeled and cut into 2-inch pieces

2 cups vegetable broth

1 teaspoon salt

½ teaspoon ground nutmeg

2 tablespoons sour cream

1. Press the Sauté button on Instant Pot. Heat 1 tablespoon olive oil. Toss turnips and carrots in oil for 1 minute. Add broth. Lock lid.
2. Press the Manual button and adjust time to 8 minutes. When timer beeps, quick release pressure until float valve drops and then unlock lid.
3. Drain vegetables and reserve liquid; set liquid aside. Add 2 tablespoons of reserved liquid plus remaining ingredients to vegetables in the Instant Pot. Use an immersion blender to blend

until desired smoothness. If too thick, add more liquid 1 tablespoon at a time. Serve warm.

Per Serving

calories: 95 | fat: 5.2g | protein: 1.4g | carbs: 11.8g | fiber: 3.0g | sodium: 669mg

Fish and Seafood

Slow Cooker Salmon in Foil

Prep time: 5 minutes | Cook time: 2 hours | Serves 2

2 (6-ounce / 170-g) salmon fillets

1 tablespoon olive oil

2 cloves garlic, minced

½ tablespoon lime juice

1 teaspoon finely chopped fresh parsley

¼ teaspoon black pepper

1. Spread a length of foil onto a work surface and place the salmon fillets in the middle.
2. Mix together the olive oil, garlic, lime juice, parsley, and black pepper in a small bowl. Brush the mixture over the fillets. Fold the foil over and crimp the sides to make a packet.
3. Place the packet into the slow cooker, cover, and cook on High for 2 hours, or until the fish flakes easily with a fork.
4. Serve hot.

Per Serving

calories: 446 | fat: 20.7g | protein: 65.4g | carbs: 1.5g | fiber: 0.2g | sodium: 240mg

Dill Chutney Salmon

Prep time: 5 minutes | Cook time: 3 minutes | Serves 2

Chutney:

¼ cup fresh dill

¼ cup extra virgin olive oil

Juice from ½ lemon

Sea salt, to taste

Fish:

2 cups water

2 salmon fillets

Juice from ½ lemon

¼ teaspoon paprika

Salt and freshly ground pepper to taste

1. Pulse all the chutney ingredients in a food processor until creamy. Set aside.
2. Add the water and steamer basket to the Instant Pot. Place salmon fillets, skin-side down, on the steamer basket. Drizzle the lemon juice over salmon and sprinkle with the paprika.
3. Secure the lid. Select the Manual mode and set the cooking time for 3 minutes at High Pressure.
4. Once cooking is complete, do a quick pressure release. Carefully open the lid.
5. Season the fillets with pepper and salt to taste. Serve topped with the dill chutney.

Per Serving

calories: 636 | fat: 41.1g | protein: 65.3g | carbs: 1.9g | fiber: 0.2g | sodium: 477mg

Garlic-Butter Parmesan Salmon and Asparagus

Prep time: 10 minutes | Cook time: 15 minutes | Serves 2

2 (6-ounce / 170-g) salmon fillets, skin on and patted dry
Pink Himalayan salt
Freshly ground black pepper, to taste

1 pound (454 g) fresh asparagus, ends snapped off
3 tablespoons almond butter
2 garlic cloves, minced
¼ cup grated Parmesan cheese

1. Preheat the oven to 400ºF (205ºC). Line a baking sheet with aluminum foil.
2. Season both sides of the salmon fillets with salt and pepper.
3. Put the salmon in the middle of the baking sheet and arrange the asparagus around the salmon.
4. Heat the almond butter in a small saucepan over medium heat.
5. Add the minced garlic and cook for about 3 minutes, or until the garlic just begins to brown.

6. Drizzle the garlic-butter sauce over the salmon and asparagus and scatter the Parmesan cheese on top.

7. Bake in the preheated oven for about 12 minutes, or until the salmon is cooked through and the asparagus is crisp-tender. You can switch the oven to broil at the end of cooking time for about 3 minutes to get a nice char on the asparagus.

8. Let cool for 5 minutes before serving.

Per Serving

calories: 435 | fat: 26.1g | protein: 42.3g | carbs: 10.0g | fiber: 5.0g | sodium: 503mg

Lemon Rosemary Roasted Branzino

Prep time: 15 minutes | Cook time: 30 minutes | Serves 2

4 tablespoons extra-virgin olive oil, divided

2 (8-ounce / 227-g) branzino fillets, preferably at least 1 inch thick

1 garlic clove, minced

1 bunch scallions (white part only), thinly sliced

10 to 12 small cherry tomatoes, halved

1 large carrot, cut into ¼-inch rounds

½ cup dry white wine

2 tablespoons paprika

2 teaspoons kosher salt

½ tablespoon ground chili pepper

2 rosemary sprigs or 1 tablespoon dried rosemary

1 small lemon, thinly sliced

½ cup sliced pitted kalamata olives

1. Heat a large ovenproof skillet over high heat until hot, about 2 minutes. Add 1 tablespoon of

olive oil and heat for 10 to 15 seconds until it shimmers.

2. Add the branzino fillets, skin-side up, and sear for 2 minutes. Flip the fillets and cook for an additional 2 minutes. Set aside.
3. Swirl 2 tablespoons of olive oil around the skillet to coat evenly.
4. Add the garlic, scallions, tomatoes, and carrot, and sauté for 5 minutes, or until softened.
5. Add the wine, stirring until all ingredients are well combined. Carefully place the fish over the sauce.
6. Preheat the oven to 450ºF (235ºC).
7. Brush the fillets with the remaining 1 tablespoon of olive oil and season with paprika, salt, and chili pepper. Top each fillet with a rosemary sprig and lemon slices. Scatter the olives over fish and around the skillet.
8. Roast for about 10 minutes until the lemon slices are browned. Serve hot.

Per Serving

calories: 724 | fat: 43.0g | protein: 57.7g | carbs: 25.0g | fiber: 10.0g | sodium: 2950mg

Grilled Lemon Pesto Salmon

Prep time: 5 minutes | Cook time: 6 to 10 minutes | Serves 2

10 ounces (283 g) salmon fillet (1 large piece or 2 smaller ones)

2 tablespoons prepared pesto sauce

Salt and freshly ground black pepper, to taste

1 large fresh lemon, sliced

Cooking spray

1. reheat the grill to medium-high heat. Spray the grill grates with cooking spray.
2. Season the salmon with salt and black pepper. Spread the pesto sauce on top.
3. Make a bed of fresh lemon slices about the same size as the salmon fillet on the hot grill, and place the salmon on top of the lemon slices. Put any additional lemon slices on top of the salmon.
4. Grill the salmon for 6 to 10 minutes, or until the fish is opaque and flakes apart easily.
5. Serve hot.

Per Serving

calories: 316 | fat: 21.1g | protein: 29.0g | carbs: 1.0g | fiber: 0g | sodium: 175mg

Steamed Trout with Lemon Herb Crust

Prep time: 10 minutes | Cook time: 15 minutes | Serves 2

3 tablespoons olive oil

3 garlic cloves, chopped

2 tablespoons fresh lemon juice

1 tablespoon chopped fresh mint

1 tablespoon chopped fresh parsley

¼ teaspoon dried ground thyme

1 teaspoon sea salt

1 pound (454 g) fresh trout (2 pieces)

2 cups fish stock

1. Stir together the olive oil, garlic, lemon juice, mint, parsley, thyme, and salt in a small bowl. Brush the marinade onto the fish.
2. Insert a trivet in the Instant Pot. Pour in the fish stock and place the fish on the trivet.
3. Secure the lid. Select the Steam mode and set the cooking time for 15 minutes at High Pressure.
4. Once cooking is complete, do a quick pressure release. Carefully open the lid. Serve warm.

Per Serving

calories: 477 | fat: 29.6g | protein: 51.7g | carbs: 3.6g | fiber: 0.2g | sodium: 2011mg

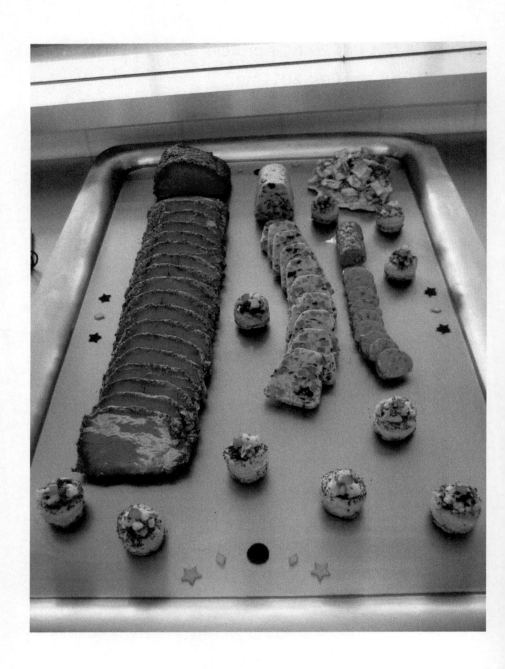

Roasted Trout Stuffed with Veggies

Prep time: 10 minutes | Cook time: 25 minutes | Serves 2

2 (8-ounce / 227-g) whole trout fillets, dressed (cleaned but with bones and skin intact)
1 tablespoon extra-virgin olive oil
¼ teaspoon salt
⅛ teaspoon freshly ground black pepper
1 small onion, thinly sliced
½ red bell pepper, seeded and thinly sliced
1 poblano pepper, seeded and thinly sliced
2 or 3 shiitake mushrooms, sliced
1 lemon, sliced
Nonstick cooking spray

1. Preheat the oven to 425ºF (220ºC). Spray a baking sheet with nonstick cooking spray.
2. Rub both trout fillets, inside and out, with the olive oil. Season with salt and pepper.
3. Mix together the onion, bell pepper, poblano pepper, and mushrooms in a large bowl. Stuff

half of this mixture into the cavity of each fillet. Top the mixture with 2 or 3 lemon slices inside each fillet.

4. Place the fish on the prepared baking sheet side by side. Roast in the preheated oven for 25 minutes, or until the fish is cooked through and the vegetables are tender.

5. Remove from the oven and serve on a plate.

Per Serving

calories: 453 | fat: 22.1g | protein: 49.0g | carbs: 13.8g | fiber: 3.0g | sodium: 356mg

Lemony Trout with Caramelized Shallots

Prep time: 10 minutes | Cook time: 20 minutes | Serves 2

Shallots:

1 teaspoon almond butter

2 shallots, thinly sliced Dash salt

Trout:

1 tablespoon plus 1 teaspoon almond butter, divided

2 (4-ounce / 113-g) trout fillets

3 tablespoons capers

¼ cup freshly squeezed lemon juice

¼ teaspoon salt

Dash freshly ground black pepper

1 lemon, thinly sliced

Make the Shallots

1. In a large skillet over medium heat, cook the butter, shallots, and salt for 20 minutes, stirring every 5 minutes, or until the shallots are wilted and caramelized. Make the Trout

2. Meanwhile, in another large skillet over medium heat, heat 1 teaspoon of almond butter.

3. Add the trout fillets and cook each side for 3 minutes, or until flaky. Transfer to a plate and set aside.

4. In the skillet used for the trout, stir in the capers, lemon juice, salt, and pepper, then bring to a simmer. Whisk in the remaining 1 tablespoon of almond butter. Spoon the sauce over the fish.

5. Garnish the fish with the lemon slices and caramelized shallots before serving.

Per Serving

calories: 344 | fat: 18.4g | protein: 21.1g | carbs: 14.7g | fiber: 5.0g | sodium: 1090mg

Tomato Tuna Melts

Prep time: 5 minutes | Cook time: 3 to 4 minutes | Serves 2

1 (5-ounce / 142-g) can chunk light tuna packed in water, drained

2 tablespoons plain Greek yogurt

2 tablespoons finely chopped celery

1 tablespoon finely chopped red onion

2 teaspoons freshly squeezed lemon juice

Pinch cayenne pepper

1 large tomato, cut into ¾-inch-thick rounds

½ cup shredded Cheddar cheese

1. Preheat the broiler to High.
2. Stir together the tuna, yogurt, celery, red onion, lemon juice, and cayenne pepper in a medium bowl.
3. Place the tomato rounds on a baking sheet. Top each with some tuna salad and Cheddar cheese.
4. Broil for 3 to 4 minutes until the cheese is melted and bubbly. Cool for 5 minutes before serving.

Per Serving

calories: 244 | fat: 10.0g | protein: 30.1g | carbs: 6.9g | fiber: 1.0g | sodium: 445mg

Mackerel and Green Bean Salad

Prep time: 10 minutes | Cook time: 10 minutes | Serves 2

2 cups green beans

1 tablespoon avocado oil

2 mackerel fillets

4 cups mixed salad greens

2 hard-boiled eggs, sliced

1 avocado, sliced

2 tablespoons lemon juice

2 tablespoons olive oil

1 teaspoon Dijon mustard

Salt and black pepper, to taste

1. Cook the green beans in a medium saucepan of boiling water for about 3 minutes until crisp-tender. Drain and set aside.
2. Melt the avocado oil in a pan over medium heat. Add the mackerel fillets and cook each side for 4 minutes.
3. Divide the greens between two salad bowls. Top with the mackerel, sliced egg, and avocado slices.
4. In another bowl, whisk together the lemon juice, olive oil, mustard, salt, and pepper, and

drizzle over the salad. Add the cooked green beans and toss to combine, then serve.

Per Serving

calories: 737 | fat: 57.3g | protein: 34.2g | carbs: 22.1g | fiber: 13.4g | sodium: 398mg